Homeopathy

Understanding Homeopathy

An Option for Your Health Care

In Epidemics, in Acute, Recurring and
Chronic Conditions
With
Emotional and Behavioral Problems

Traudl Woehlke

Series Whole Health Now Vol. II

ISBN 978-1542728119

Manufactured in the United States of America

Sundance-Verlag
Kaiserstr. 32
68766 Hockenheim

"Homeopathy is one of the few medical specialities which carries no penalties – only benefits." –Yehudi Menuhin

According to the WHO, homeopathy is the fastest growing medicine worldwide. Also in the United States, a new interest in homeopathy has emerged. Homeopathy has been wildly successful in gently treating and preventing severe epidemics, infections, chronic disease and everyday ills, even plant and animal disease. Its successes have been recorded since its first origins in 1796. Homeopathy has been a revolutionary and unique system of medicine from its very beginnings, and to date we have not yet fully discovered why it works. We do know, however, how to apply and use it for our own good.

This book was written to help you understand homeopathy in short - what homeopathy is all about and what it can do for you, when you are considering homeopathy as an option for your health care, HOMEOPATHY: UNDERSTANDING HOMEOPATHY AND WHAT IT CAN DO FOR YOU provides you with all the details you need to know for an informed decision.

To your health!

About the Author

Traudl Woehlke is a German licensed healing practitioner specializing in homeopathy, whole and raw food nutrition, and energy psychology (tapping).

Message from the Author

Health is a matter of being informed!

No one but yourself is interested in your personal health as there is big money being made with disease. This is the main reason why you find so much confusing and contradictory health information in the media and on the internet.

It is my passion to provide you with the hidden knowledge it takes to regain and maintain health and to encourage and empower you to take control of your health and well-being.

Best,

Traudl Woehlke

Table of Contents

Chapter 1 - What is Homeopathy?

"Homeopathy is one of the few medical specialities which carries no penalties – only benefits." –Yehudi Menuhin

Introduction

Have you ever crushed a finger? It sure hurts and takes a long time to heal. Well, my first personal experience with homeopathy was the cure of a crushed finger – a horse had chewed my finger which quickly doubled in width and hurt terribly. (Don't ask why my finger got into the horse's mouth – I thought the horse would suck my hand like a young calf, so I left my finger in its mouth until the horse started to chew on it!) About an hour later I could get ahold of the homeopathic remedy Arnica and took some of those tiny pillules. Within 30 minutes, the terrible pain in my finger was gone for good. The finger kept its normal color and did not turn black or blue as you would expect, and after a few days the swelling was gone too. This was quite impressive, and the beginning of my serious interest in homeopathy. Since then, I got an education in homeopathy, and I have practiced homeopathy for nearly 15 years, with impressive results in humans and animals.

I invite you to discover how you too can benefit from homeopathy.

Let's look and see what homeopathy is and what it isn't as there exists a lot of confusion about the term "homeopathy".

When searching for treatment options on the internet, in health food stores, in self-help books, and when talking to a friend for a home remedy, the term "Homeopathy" pops up. If you ask a conventional doctor for a non-prescription drug, he may prescribe "something homeopathic" to you.

Well, it isn't home remedies, herbs, or naturopathy, or a harmless drug.

Homeopathy Defined

Homeopathy is a powerful scientific system of medicine based on the universal law of similar meaning like cures like. It is radically different from any other system of medicine, and has been proven effective, and gentle since 1796 all over the world. Homeopathy is used on every continent to treat humans, animals and plants with impressive results in acute and even severe chronic conditions, and in epidemics

When homeopathy is practiced at its highest standards, it is the treatment of choice to recover one's health from the great majority of acute and chronic diseases.

Homeopathy treats sick people with remedies that would produce in healthy people symptoms similar to those of the disease needing to be overcome. This is the application of the universal law of similar.

The Law of Similar

Even if you have never heard of the law of similar, you most likely are familiar with its effect. For example, when you chop a red onion, pretty soon you will have burning tears streaming, and a watery runny nose. These are some of the symptoms onions cause in a healthy person. When you have a condition with symptoms of a watery runny nose and burning streaming eyes (such as in hay fever or a cold) similar to what you get from cutting an onion, the homeopathic remedy allium cepa (onion) corresponds to your condition and is the curative homeopathic remedy.

This is exactly what homeopathy does: the curative homeopathy medicine will be one that matches in detail the characteristic symptoms the patient is suffering from.

Symptoms

Your symptoms are essential for finding the curative homeopathic remedy. They are considered signals of your system asking for a particular stimulus to trigger your natural defense mechanism/immunity (vital force) to do the healing.

For cure, symptoms need to be overcome by your body's healing forces. The well-chosen homeopathic remedy triggers your body to do its own healing.

If symptoms are suppressed, they tend to return in disguise in a form worse than before. For instance, many times asthma occurs after skin symptoms have been suppressed by topical treatment.

Once a health problem is overcome naturally in the way indicated above, as a result not only will the symptoms disappear, also your overall health will be at a higher level than before the illness.

Homeopathic Remedies

Homeopathic remedies often times are diluted, and they all are prepared in a special way to unfold their curative effects. This makes homeopathy one of the most gentle and most safe medicines there is.

The Origin of Homeopathy

"The highest aim of healing is the rapid, gentle, and permanent restitution of health ... in the shortest, most reliable, and safest manner, according to clearly intelligible reasons." -Samuel Hahnemann, M.D.

Homeopathy was founded by the physician Samuel Hahnemann (1755 – 1843). He was both a medical doctor and pharmacist, and a chemist.

Hahnemann was a very intelligent man way ahead of his time and age. As a child, he was already fluent in several foreign languages. While in med school, he earned his living as a scientific translator. As a doctor, he soon was disillusioned with medical practice of his day, and he quit practicing. He went into research instead, and continued translating English, French, and Italian texts.

When he translated works of the London professor of medicine William Cullen, Hahnemann learnt about the application of the cinchona bark in malaria treatment. Hahnemann wasn't satisfied with Cullen's explanations, and ingested some of the bark himself as a healthy person. He found himself with malaria symptoms after he had taken the malaria medicine. Get this: A medicine which cures a disease causes symptoms of the disease to be overcome!

This was a revolutionary discovery. Hahnemann called his trial a proving. He continued his research and tested many more substances on himself, his family and kids and on healthy volunteers.

To prevent toxic effects and In order to reduce the initial aggravation of the substance in a proving, he decreased the quantity of the test substance and diluted it more and more. At some point, no more effects could be obtained.

Hahnemann was a genius as he not only diluted the medicine, he also potentized it. Potentizing means vigorously shaking which rendered amazing effects. He resumed medical practice only after he had discovered and observed the laws of homeopathy.

Hahnemann carefully documented his procedures, methods and his results. After six years of intense research he published his findings in 1796, which was to become the birthday of homeopathy. In 1810. he published "Organon der rationellen Heilkunde", the "bible" of homeopathy. 54 of his journals dating 1800 - 1843 have been saved. They testify his very accurate and individual treatment.

Hahnemann was very much attacked when he first published his findings. Homeopathy gained wide popularity when it cured severe epidemics rampant at that time.

At 80, Hahnemann married Melanie, a young French woman and moved to Paris and became a celebrated and successful doctor.

How is Homeopathy Different from all Other Systems of Medicine?

Homeopathy is a truly holistic approach to health; it recognizes that each person responds uniquely to the forces of their heredity and environment.

So how is the homeopathic approach different from all other systems of medicine?

Example

Someone has polyps in their nose. You cut it and they grow back next year. You come back for surgery again – cut it, and they will grow back. Why?

There is a tendency within the system wanting to express that problem.

Homeopathy says the body does the best it can, and when it creates a symptom, a problem, a complaint, that's the best it can do under an adverse circumstance. This is a statement unique in all of medicine.

By creating that problem, the problem is actually a message the homeopath finds and works with. It is looked upon as a communication from our system asking for a particular stimulus.

So in homeopathy, if you have nasal polyps, the stomach aches, if you have hot feet in bed at night, your food cravings, how your moods have altered since you became unwell, all of this is one thing to the homeopath.

All of it is a message that we need to match to a medicine from nature, that when we can find that exquisite match from nature, we use the law of similar - like cures like.

So if we can get that exquisite resonating match, it will trigger in the system somewhere deep a healing that will help those problems heal themselves. So you don't need to go back, you don't need to keep taking the drugs, if we can find that exquisite match.

If we can match exactly what the body wants not only will the problem go away, but as a result the entire level of health of a human being will get better.

That's the basis of homeopathy.

Chapter 2 – Homeopathic Remedies

"The introduction of homeopathy forced the old school doctor to stir around and learn something of a rational nature about his business ..." –Mark Twain

Homeopathic remedies are prepared by licensed homeopathic pharmaceutical manufacturers derived from natural sources. They are approved by the FDA. Many substances are poisonous, so they are diluted. Their unique method of preparation makes them non-toxic, and they do not cause any side effects, yet bring out remarkable healing capacities within each individual substance.

Homeopathic remedies are available at a fraction of the cost of most prescription and over-the-counter drugs.

A large body of scientific research is proving the potent biological action of homeopathic preparations.

How are homeopathic remedies made?

Potentization

Potentization refers to the preparation of a homeopathic remedy. Each is prepared by a controlled process of successive (serial) dilutions alternating with succussion (vigorous shaking) which may be continued to the point where the resulting medicine contains no molecules of the original substance.

The more you dilute and succuss a remedy, the more effective it becomes provided it is done in this way.

Here is how you do it:

Soluble substances are dissolved in alcohol to make a "mother tincture". One part of this tincture is added to 99 parts of alcohol and succussed (vigorously shaken) at least ten times. Succussion somehow transfers the healing power of the remedy into the liquid. The result is a 1C potency (one part per hundred).

This process of serial dilution and succussion is repeated. Each step is generating a more dilute but more potent remedy. When you repeat this process ten times, you get a 10C potency, repeated one hundred times, the result is a 100C potency and so on.

The dilution can be applied in water, on tiny sugar pillules, in tablet form or a drop can be placed on a small bit of milk sugar.

Insoluble substances are triturated (ground up) with lactose for one hour using mortar and pestle. One part substance to 99 parts lactose (milk sugar) results in a 1C potency. Serial trituration is continued as described above for the higher potencies. After several serial triturations the mixture is now soluble, and the serial dilution can continue with alcohol.

Sometimes remedies are made on a decimal scale. Serial succussion or trituration for an X potency uses one part substance in 9 parts alcohol or lactose.

Potencies

These small doses are called potencies. Lesser dilutions are known as low potencies. The higher the dilution when prepared in this manner, the greater the potency of the medicine.

A potentized remedy does not contain sufficient matter to act directly on the tissue. This means a homeopathic medicine is non-toxic and cannot cause side effects. In over 200 years of use, no homeopathic remedy has ever been recalled.

Remedies Are More Than Mere Dilutions.

Homeopathic remedies are not mere dilutions. Trituration and succussion somehow intensify the potency of the source substance. The more you success a remedy, the more powerful it gets.

The process of potentization makes it possible to use substances such as certain metals, charcoal and sand, which are inert in their natural state, and poisonous substances as medicines.

How Are the Curative Effects of a Substance Discovered? (Provings)

Primarily, the range of homeopathic remedies is investigated by "proving" the substance.

Provings are single and double-blinded experiments which yield the knowledge of the action of remedies. To prove a substance, small doses are given to healthy volunteer subjects who later record their detailed reactions to the test substance.

As homeopathically prepared remedies are not toxic, there is no concern about testing homeopathic remedies on healthy individuals.

In addition, case histories of treatment with medicines that have not undergone a proving but which have yielded a cure in clinical practice have been added to the knowledge base.

Finally, the information of symptoms produced by accidental poisonings with toxic substances is added.

All those data - the provings, and clinical and toxicological data – are collected in the materia medica of the remedy. The materia medica is a reference list of the symptoms of homeopathic remedies.

To treat a patient, the homeopath looks up the remedy picture in the materia medica, and when the symptoms fit, applies the law of similar.

Safe, but Why Effective?

It's true, we do not fully know how homeopathic remedies work but we do have a recorded case history of 220 years and know from experience how to use homeopathy effectively. This is no different than with many pharmaceutical drugs which are being used even if no one knows how exactly they work.

Aspirin is just one example – it has been in use since 1899, and only in 1970 it was fully discovered how it works.

There is a lot of recent research that confirms the homeopathic approach both in laboratory tests with cell cultures and in comparing the curative results with patients and in plants. Even Darwin is known to have observed the effects of homeopathy in plants. He never published it because taking a stand for homeopathy would have been unfavorable for his own career.

Some critics blame homeopathy for its high dilutions. They insist that high dilutions cannot work as no molecules can be found in them. Science has come up with interesting research regarding the effects of high dilutions and potentization.

Professor Luc Montagnier, French virologist and Nobel laureate says: "What I can say now is that high dilutions are right. High dilutions of something are not nothing. They are water structures that mimic the original molecules. It's not pseudo-science. It's not quackery. These are real phenomena which deserve further studies."

Researchers in Brazil, Italy and India show that homeopathy is also found to work in animals and plants, apart from humans. Independent studies by scientists like molecular biologist Dr AR Khuda-Bukhsha (india), Dr Leoni Bonamin, (Brazil), Dr Paolo Bellavite (Iltaly), Dr Gaurisankar Sa (india) proved that homeopathic medicines work even on cell-line models

Read more at http://rtn.asia/d-r/10933/is-homeopathy-effective-and-safe-yes-says-practitioners-from-across-the-globe#xB5fOK1dUekMuAd3.99

Nano technology research discovered that the more a remedy is succussed, the more nano particles are created. This might explain why high potencies have a stronger effect than low potencies.

More research is needed and done to fully discover how homeopathy works.

If you still doubt, if potentization really does have an effect, go ahead and do a little simple experiment.

Take some common green bean seeds and divide them into two groups. In the first group (your control group) water them as normal. In the second group, your test group, water them as well but only after adding 5 pillules of potentized kitchen salt (Natrium-muriaticum 6C) per 50 ml or 1/2 cup water. You should see the beans from your test group grow more quickly and profusely than the control group even though a 6C potency is indistinguishable from plain water.

You can buy the Natrium-muriaticum 6C in any homeopathic pharmacy or make it yourself using table salt.

Green beans are not the only plants you can experiment with – any plant can be affected by a homeopathic potency as Darwin himself discovered.

Why Is There so Much Criticism of Homeopathy in the Media Recently?

Some media are operating on a double standard regarding homeopathy when they reiterate that homeopathy cannot work because the remedies contain no molecules. They disregard the evidence of successful cure of millions of people all over the world over a period of 220 years, and its use with plants and animals.

They also disregard all the recent research, studies and testimonials of success that exist.

This is not new. Throughout history, homeopathy has been attacked and oppressed because of its success which is a real potential threat to conventional medicine and the pharmaceutical industry. Whenever homeopathy was getting popular, it was perceived as a threat to the business of mainstream medicine and its associated industries.

It's been lay people who have educated themselves in the application of homeopathy and got organized in homeopathic lay groups. They helped homeopathy survive by preserving the interest in homeopathy, and experience and knowledge.

The links provide you with a list of evidence based research on homeopathy:

http://www.britishhomeopathic.org/wp-content/uploads/2013/05/evidencesummary.pdf

http://hpathy.com/scientific-research/database-of-positive-homeopathy-research-studies/

Chapter 3 - Historical Background

"You may honestly feel grateful that homeopathy survived the attempts of the allopaths to destroy it." - Mark Twain

Hahnemann was scorned by many of his contemporaries as you may imagine as it was a radically different kind of approach.

Homeopathy first gained a huge following in Europe through its effective treatment and prevention of cholera, typhoid, measles, scarlet and yellow fever with a mortality rate of 3 - 6 % or less without any side effects as to 30 to 70% mortality of conventional medicine.

Dr. Constantin Hering, a German immigrant, founded the first homeopathic medical school in the United States in 1844.

Just like in Europe, homeopathy gained recognition because of its success in treating the many disease epidemics raging at the time — including scarlet fever, typhoid, cholera and yellow fever. In the mid-1850s, patients were leaving orthodox doctors in droves to be treated by homeopathy.

Homeopathy became very popular in the early 1900's. At that time, there were 22 homeopathic medical schools, 100 homeopathic hospitals and over 1,000 homeopathic pharmacies. Boston University, Stanford University and New York Medical College were among those educational institutions that were teaching homeopathy.

However, already in the 1920s many of those medical schools closed.

Homeopathy lost its popularity in the United States mostly for three reasons:

1. Modern drug companies began releasing drugs such as penicillin that were easy to administer to patients.

2. The American Medical Association (AMA) was formed in 1847 with the declared purpose of destroying homeopathy. It funded its activities by granting seals of approval to any synthetic drug that advertised in its journal.

3. The homeopaths were a divided profession. They did not stand together as one to counteract .the negative trends. Also quite a few so-called homeopaths did not follow the rules of homeopathy, and many were poorly trained.

While the United States experienced a declining interest in homeopathy in the 20th century, other nations, including countries in Europe and Asia, were experiencing a steady growth of homeopathic teachings and interest.

Recent Development: Homeopathy is the World's Fastest Growing Medicine

In the United States, since 1970 public interest has risen again, and homeopathy is coming back in North America.

Americans spent 230 million dollars on homeopathic remedies in 1996. It has also been said that sales are rising rapidly at about 12 – 15% each year.

Meanwhile it is used all over the world to treat humans, animals and plants with impressive results in acute and even severe chronic conditions.

Homeopathy in the World

Today, all French and German pharmacies sell homeopathic remedies. In France, 30% of all physicians prescribe homeopathic medicines, 20% in Germany, and 40% in the UK.

Homeopathy has been integrated into the healthcare systems of many countries including France, Germany, the Netherlands, Italy, Switzerland, Brazil and Portugal. It is popular in Russia, Switzerland, France, Italy, Germany, Netherlands, England, Argentina and Mexico, India, Pakistan and Sri Lanka.

Mahatma Gandhi promoted homeopathy in India where it is recognized as one of the three pillars of public medicine together with Ayurveda and Western medicine.

In Germany, med students must take at least one introductory course in homeopathy. The German agricultural department sponsors courses in homeopathy for farmers to enable them to treat their animals without antibiotics.

Homeopathy and Epidemics

Homeopathy has been a viable alternative to standard medicine for over 220 years. Governments of today are using homeopathy to prevent, treat, or break epidemics within their countries. Homeopathy is a safe alternative to vaccinations which all come with health risk. To learn how to naturally prevent virus infections, please get "Vaccine-free Healthy in a Viral Epidemic".

Some examples of recent homeopathic epidemics mastery are:

- The Indian government controls epidemics of malaria, Japanese encephalitis, dengue fever, and epidemic fever with homeopathy

- The Cuban government now depends on the homeopathic preparation of medicines to manage its leptospirosis epidemics and dengue fever outbreaks.

- The Brazilian government funded two large trials that successfully reduced the incidence of meningococcal disease in those given the homeopathic prophylactic.

- The governments of Thailand, Colombo and Brazil use homeopathy to manage dengue fever outbreaks and epidemics.
  http://homeopathyplus.com.au/Homeoprophylaxis-Human-Records-Studies-Trials.pdf

- In 2014, homeopaths have successfully cured Ebola patients in Africa as reported by John Benneth.

Chapter 4 - Why Use Homeopathy?

"Homeopathy is wholly capable of satisfying the therapeutic demands of this age better than any other system or school of medicine." – C. F. Menninger MD (Founder of the Menninger Clinic)

Below is a list of benefits.

- Homeopathy works. As long as the remedy is well chosen.

- Homeopathy treats the whole person. This allows corresponding and seemingly unrelated issues to fall away as well.

- Homeopathy has no side effects.

- Homeopathy is not addictive.

- Homeopathy is safe even for the unborn child.

- Homeopathy is approved by the FDA and unlike modern drugs, has never had a history of even one remedy having been forced off the market for adverse reactions.

- Homeopathy is inexpensive.

- Homeopathy works with nature, not against nature.

- Homeopathy has 220 years of double blind data to support its claims.

- Homeopathy works on children, infants, the elderly, plants, pets and livestock.

- Homeopathy is building the next generation stronger physically and emotionally.

- Homeopathy can be lifesaving, and it can also remove mild pain and deal with everyday ills as well.

- Homeopathy is easy to dispense.

- Even lay persons can learn to apply homeopathy.

- Homeopathic remedies can last a VERY long time if stored correctly.

- Homeopathy has reduced environmental impact: fewer chemicals involved in producing the drugs

- Homeopathy avoids supporting the corporations that are linked to chemical manufacturers (and GMO crops).

Who Has Used Homeopathy?

In general, people using homeopathy tend to be better educated and better informed persons than those going for conventional (allopathic) medicine.

Homeopathy has a reputation for being preferred by the privileged and famous. These are the people who could afford to select any medicine in the world, yet depended on homeopathy.

Famous people who used homeopathy include Abraham Lincoln, Tina Turner, Sir Paul McCartney, Charles Darwin, the violinist Paganini, John D. Rockefeller (who lived 99 years), three American presidents, and Bill Clinton, Daniel Webster, former prime minister Tony Blair, Henry W. Longfellow, Washington Irving, Nathaniel Hawthorne, Harriet Beecher Stowe, Florence Nightingale, Mahatma Gandhi, P. Nehru, Mark Twain, Samuel Morse, Yehudi Menuhin, a great part of the aristocracy and European royalty. The British Royal Family, a number of popes including Pius X, John Paul II, and Benedict XVI. Also Mother Teresa's Mission of Charity applies homeopathy.

Chapter 5 - How to Take a Remedy

"I also turn to Homeopathic remedies for the treatment of indigestion, travel sickness, insomnia and hay fever just to name a few. Homeopathy offers a safe, natural alternative that causes no side effects or drug interactions" –Cindy Crawford

The Single Remedy – Only One Remedy at a Time

In classical homeopathy as taught by Hahnemann, usually only one remedy at a time is taken. This is in contrast to the current medical practice of frequently prescribing two or more medicines.

After the remedy is given, its action is assessed some time later. If it is working no more medicine is given unless the improvements experienced either stop completely or are reversed. If symptoms shift, a new remedy needs to be found to match the recent symptoms.

No combinations of medicines are given as combination medicines have not been proved in their particular combination. We are not sure what the effect of a particular combination would be in a healthy person nor do we know what the interaction between those remedies would be. But we are sure of the effect of a single remedy which lets us assess the process of healing in an individual.

The Minimum Dose

The best results are obtained by taking the minimum amount of medicinal stimulus to get a reaction from your own healing powers.

Currently, you find much misinformation relating to repetition and dosage of homeopathic medicines, both on the medicine containers and in magazine articles and self-help books. Ignore any instructions that ask you to routinely repeat a homeopathic medicine at set intervals. Do not repeat a remedy as long as improvement continues.

What Else to Consider

There are some substance that antidote homeopathic medicines. An antidote neutralizes the effects of another substance. In the case of homeopathy, the administered remedy would become ineffective by the antidote.

Substances to avoid are caffeine/coffee, coke, mint, camphor, menthol, eucalyptus, and chamomile topically or ingested.

To avoid camphor, menthol, and eucalyptus, you need to read the labels of your home remedies and ointments to make sure you are not erroneously getting some (such as tiger balm).

- One dose is 3-5 pillules (pillules are those little white sugar balls that are medicated with the remedy.)

- Avoid eating approximately 20-30 minutes before and after taking remedies for best results. This is what most homeopaths recommend. In my experience with treating animals, eating does not interfere with the action of remedies. In fact, I add remedies to the food of an animal if I cannot give it straight into its mouth.

- In an acute injury or ill, you may need to initially repeat the remedy very frequently – as much as every 3 minutes. Stop taking it whenever you experience the slightest improvement. Continue when you feel the remedy is no longer working.

- If you need to take 2 different remedies, space your dosages out over the course of the day, with no less than 60 minutes in between different remedies.
    - Example: Two different remedies are to be taken twice daily. Remedy No. 1 can be taken at 8AM and 4PM and remedy No. 2 can be taken at 11AM and 8PM.
- A strong physical or emotional shock, sudden grief or major surgery may interrupt the course of a "running" remedy. In this case, you need to address the respective issue first with the appropriate remedy before continuing with the original treatment. (Homeopathy is excellent in supporting healing in surgery and post-operative care.)

There are several ways to take a remedy

Method 1: Taking the Remedy as it is

- Take 2 or 3 pillules or one tablet as they are into your mouth and let them dissolve.
- If you are taking a tincture, you may dilute 2 or 3 drops in a teaspoon of water. Keep the fluid in your mouth as long as you can.

If you need to administer the homeopathic medicine to an unconscious or sleeping person, or an animal, you can just put it into their mouth.

Method 2: Taking the Remedy Dissolved in Water

You need a clean glass of water, and a spoon for vigorously stirring. (Some homeopaths recommend to use plastic cups and plastic spoons which have to be discharged after use.) When using a glass and a metal spoon, they need to be cleaned in the dishwasher or boiled in hot water before re-using them for homeopathic remedies.

- Add 2 – 6 pillules or drops of a tincture to the water.
- Stir to dissolve.
- Take a teaspoon or a small sip of the fluid.
- Stir briskly every time before you take another dose of the diluted medicine.
- Cover it with a saucer between doses. Your remedy will be fine to use in this manner for one or two days. To preserve it for about a week, add a tablespoon of brandy to the water.

Method 3 Sniffing (Olfaction Dosing)

Remedies can also be taken through the nose by a quick sniff. It's called olfaction dosing.

In olfaction dosing the energy of remedy is taken inward with a quick breath. It has been in use since the early days of homeopathy. It is ideally suited for sensitive people who overreact to oral doses.

- Place one or two pillules of the remedy in a vial or small bottle.
- Hold this container close to your nose as you take an inward breath.
- You can take the same approach for remedies in liquid form. Simply hold the open bottle under your nose when inhaling.
- Inhaling by mouth works just as well.

Hahnemann is reported to have been refused pay when he had administered olfaction dosing to a patient. Instead of handing the due pay to Hahnemann, the patient offered to let him sniff the money! This may be the reason why sniffing is not in wide use.

How long does it take until I see improvement with homeopathy?

In acute conditions, you can expect quick results with homeopathy. First improvement usually can be felt within 15 to 60 minutes after taking the remedy, provided it is matching your symptoms. If you do not feel any change in your condition after having taken the remedy, you may take it 2 or 3 more times even in a different potency. If there is still no reaction, you need to find a better matching remedy.

It is different with chronic conditions which generally are more complex to treat. Their cure may take quite some time. Usually first signs of improvements can be felt in your mood.

Chapter 6 – The Scope of Homeopathy

"Homeopathy cures a larger percentage of cases than any other method of treatment and is beyond doubt safer and more economical and the most complete medical system." – *Mahatma Gandhi*

Homeopathy in Acute, Recurring and Chronic Conditions

Homeopathy has been used to treat and prevent disease in humans, animals, and plants. Homeopathy cures acute conditions and recurring illnesses such as the tendency of bronchitis or urinary infections, and allergies. Many stubborn and severe chronic conditions have been cured. If cure is not possible, homeopathy provides pain relief.

Homeopathy is the most frequently used complementary therapy in pediatric oncology in Germany.

Homeopathy in Infectious Diseases and Epidemics

Homeopathy has a long recorded history of successful preventing and curing infectious diseases and epidemics such as the flu, polio, cholera, hepatitis, encephalitis, dengue fever, yellow fever, leptospirosis, malaria, to name a few.

Unlike vaccination shots and anti-viral meds, homeopathy comes without side effects, and costs only a fraction of conventional drugs. It can be given to the newborn and in old age and to animals and plants.

This is especially important to know after in August 2014, a "whistle-blower" of the American governmental Center for

Disease Control and Prevention (CDC), a respected PhD scientist, claimed the CDC 'hid' the findings of a 2002 study which linked the MMR vaccine to a 340% increase in autism among African-American children.

Interesting, the mainstream media did not report it, and you could learn about it only via the internet and alternative media. Here is the link to find out more.

http://www.naturalnews.com/046614_CDC_whistleblower _vaccine_cover-up_criminal_investigation.html

Homeopathy for all stages of life

Homeopathy in Pregnancy, Childbirth, Infancy and Childhood

It is completely safe in treating pregnant women, infants and children.
Homeopathy addresses fertility issues, pregnancy problems including miscarriages, eases childbirth and delivery, cures mastitis, and can be given to the newborn. Many expectant mothers have been able to avoid Caesarean section with homeopathy. Many times breech children (those that are positioned bottom down in the womb) have altered this position to head-down which allowed a regular natural birth with the help of the remedy Pulsatilla.

Childhood developmental issues, behavioral disorders, ADD/ADHS and autism are within the scope of homeopathy. Also childhood diseases, eczema, allergies, asthma respond to homeopathic treatment. Fevers, colds, ear infections, diarrhea, vomiting, sore throat, teething pain can be addressed with the matching homeopathic remedies. A strep throat responds well to Hepar sulfuris 200C. Teething pain is eased with Chamomilla 30C, ear ache frequently is cured with Pulsatilla.

Homeopathy in Women's Health

Women benefit from homeopathy with menstrual disorders, pregnancy and menopause problems, cysts, polyps and fibroids. Breast illnesses, and endometriosis, and infections of female organs.

Homeopathy in the Treatment of Stroke, Heart Attack, Inflammation, Musculoskeletal Diseases

Homeopathy has been successful in treating stroke and heart attacks, back pain, inflammation, joint problems such as frozen shoulder, sciatica, osteoarthritis, rheumatoid arthritis, migraines, headache.

Homeopathy in Other Civilatory Diseases

The symptoms of diabetes, thyroid disturbances, skin diseases, even psoriasis, and vitiligo, nasal polyps, colitis, digestive issues, and allergies, disease of the nervous system as neuritis, multiple sclerosis have been treated with well-chosen homeopathic remedies.

Homeopathy in Old Age

In old age, homeopathy has been used for palliative care and pain relief in incurable conditions. Many care takers have experienced an easier burden when the old person receives homeopathic treatment which quiets them without numbing by tranquilizers. It has improved the symptoms of dementia and the progression of Alzheimer's. The main remedy for dementia is Helleborus 30C.

Also, it helps the bed-ridden old person to cough up and expec-torate mucus without need for suction. The remedy is Antimonium tartaricum 30C.

Homeopathy for the Dying

Homeopathy can also be beneficial when dying. It helps the per-son to let go without fear.

Homeopathy in First Aid

Homeopathy is excellent for treating injuries, and in first aid and shock it may be lifesaving when you give it immediately even if you need to call the ambulance. By the time the physician arrives, the right remedy may have improved the condition of the injured person already. Typically the first remedy with injuries is Arnica which absorbs bruises in soft tissues. Incase of shock conditions, Aconitum will quickly do away with it.

Homeopathy in Surgery and Dentistry

In surgery and dental treatment, homeopathy speeds healing, recovery and reliefs pain. When combined with surgery, you can expect healing without scars. It removes adhesions, prevents infection of wounds and heals burns.

It can cure shock conditions, resolve trauma, new and old grief, home sickness and emotional distress. New grief requires Ignatia 30C, old grief calls for Natrium chloratum 30C or 200C.

Dental conditions commonly seen by homeopathic dentists are apical abscess, anxiety, tooth extraction, sensitive cementum, periodontal abscess, post-surgery pain, gum swelling, reversible pulpitis, toothache with decay, periodontitis. Periodontal abscesses respond to Hepar sulfuris 30C, Mercurius solubilis 200C has been used to cure gum bleeding.

Homeopathy for Psychological Disorders, Mental Health and People with Behavior Problems (Autism, ADHD, Depression)

From its very beginnings, homeopathy has helped and cured people with mental and psychiatric problems. It is still effective with mental and behavioral problems today.

Homeopathy given while under psychotherapy, improves the treatment results considerably in shorter time.

In general, fears, phobias including social phobias, obsessional neuroses, disturbances in learning, ADHS in children, depression and many other mental illnesses respond well to homeopathic treatment. Depression in men frequently calls for Aurum 200C, in women, Sepia 200C often will be curative.

Homeopathy has helped to overcome addiction.

The homeopathic Swiss pediatrician Dr. Heiner Frei, MD, has fine-tuned the treatment of ADHD in children, and when done with the right homeopathic methods, the success rate is around 70% - without any side effects for the child.

Dr. Heiner Frei has conducted the now famous Berne ADS/ADHS Double Blind Study from 2000 to 2005. The study was consistent with strict standards of conventional medicine and has proven the efficiency of homeopathy as a scientific method.

Homeopathy is reported to be effective in the treatment of autism too. You can find many case stories on the internet for details. The treatment of autism takes a lot longer than the treatment of ADHS.

Homeopathy for Animals and Plants

Homeopaths have treated animals both farmed animals and pets, even birds, fish in a tank, and turtles.

Agro-homeopathy is used to treat plant diseases and improve soil conditions and growth and to balance unfavorable climate and weather effects. It also works for pests control such as slug and snails. For details please see the following chapter.

Homeopathy in Cancer Treatment

Indian homeopaths are experienced in treating cancer and other very serious conditions with remarkable success.

The Swiss homeopathic hospital Clinica Santa Croce in Orsellina, reports a 30% success rate in the treatment of cancer patients who have been given up by conventional medicine. Those who cannot be cured get palliative relief from the disease and the side effects of chemo and radiation therapy.

37

(Conventional medicine considers a therapy with a 30% success rate as successful. The homeopaths of Santa Croce achieve this rate with patients who are considered untreatable by standard medicine.)

This list is by no means exhaustive.

For testimonials, visit the website "Homeopathy worked for me".

Can Homeopathy Cure All Disease Conditions?

The answer is no.

Homeopathy can effectively help with those conditions in which there is no irreversible pathology. If an organ has been destroyed such as a joint with chronic osteoarthritis, or a cavity in a tooth, homeopathy cannot restore the original condition of the body. Only palliative care is possible. This still has its benefits over conventional pain killers as homeopathy comes without side effects.

Homeopathy cannot replace surgery. In surgery it has its place as it promotes recovery and healing and prevents the formation of scars and adhesions. Existing adhesions can be reversed.

Homeopathy stimulates the vital force of an individual. If the vital force is too weak to respond as at the end of life, in terminal stages of cancer or other severe diseases or if it has been damaged by the use of drugs, or conventional medicine, an individual may not respond to homeopathy.

Some conditions are very difficult to treat. Most likely, homeopathy can offer relief without side effects.

Chapter 7 –Plant Disease and Pest Control With Homeopathy

"Homeopathic doses are perhaps the strongest" –Feodor Dostoevsky

Literally anything that is alive can benefit from homeopathic treatment, be it plants, animals or human beings. So if slugs and snails are eating your vegetables, your roses are afflicted with lice, voles destroy the roots of your vegetables, mildew affects your flowers, grapes and pumpkins, blight becomes a problem, homeopathy can fight and prevent them without poison. Also fungal, bacterial and viral plant infections can be cured and prevented with the corresponding homeopathic remedies.

Homeopathy can improve the effects of unfavorable weather effects such as drought, too much rain, late frosts and cold.

And there are remedies to improve the growth and flavor of tomatoes.

In general, just like humans, also plants respond with an increase of general health and better strength to homeopathic treatment. Strong healthy plants reward the gardener with better crops.

Best of all, those remedies are inexpensive, so you can enjoy organic garden produce at low cost.

Surprisingly, there exists a wide range of experience in the homeopathic treatment of plants in many countries. It's not just hobby gardeners, also professional farmers and vine growers manage plant and soil health with homeopathy.

The Second International Conference on Homeopathy for Plants was held in Maringa, Brazil in September 2013.

Modern research in agro homeopathy is done in New Zealand, Australia, Chile, Italy, Spain, Latin America, Africa, India, Pakistan and the Middle East, UK, USA, Switzerland, Brazil, Mexico and Cuba.

If you are a home gardener, this book is for you:

http://www.amazon.com/Homeopathy-Plants-practical-balcony-potency/dp/3943309215/ref=sr_1_1?s=books&ie=UTF8&qid=1427799166&s

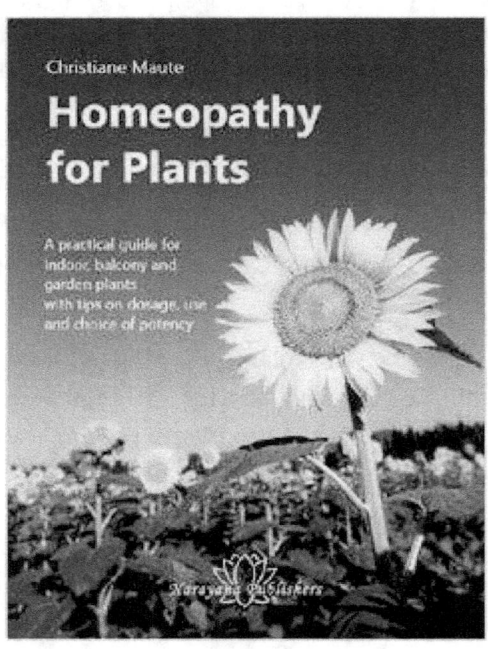

Chapter 8 - Who Practices Homeopathy?

"If I was not an actress, I would be a homeopathic doctor." – Lindsay Wagner

Homeopaths can be medical doctors, and in the United States, many homeopaths are also chiropractors, naturopaths, osteopaths, nurse practitioners, dentists and veterinarians.

There also are many unlicensed homeopathic practitioners. They usually are persons without an accredited medical education or live in a state that does not allow licensing of homeopathy.

In the United States, state law regulates the licensing of medical professions.

The skills and experience of homeopaths vary. Some start practicing after a few introductory courses, others start only after many years of training.

How to Find a Good Homeopath

There are homeopathic practitioners who are medical doctors and those who are not licensed as a medically trained practitioner.

The best way to find a good homeopath is a referral by a happy patient.

Or you may call the practitioners in your area and find out if they are classical and how much time they allow for the first visit. They should allow a minimum of one hour and not work with combination remedies.

Another way is to call a homeopathic study group in your area and ask them. You can find a study group in your area in the referral list of the National Center for Homeopathy.

http://www.nationalcenterforhomeopathy.org/

If you are looking for a qualified homeopath, here is what you may want to find out:

1. What is his experience and training, and any testimonials.
   With medically licensed homeopaths, find out what the proportion of homeopathic treatment is in his practice. He should specialize in homeopathy as the primary therapy.

2. How much time is allowed for a first visit, and what type of remedies are prescribed. If combination remedies are applied, this is not classical homeopathy as outlined in this book. You cannot expect the same benefits as with classical (single remedy) homeopathy

There is a list of links of homeopathic associations with listed members in the last section of this book.

Chapter 9 - What To Expect in a Homeopathic Consultation

"We are at a turning point in medical history, when, having recognized the outer limits of technological medicine, doctors and lay people are together discovering the vast powers for creating health that we each inherit at birth." — Hal Zina Bennet

Homeopathic doctors work in the same way as conventional doctors do. History taking, examination and investigation are all important in establishing the diagnosis.

In addition, a homeopath will also be interested in you as an individual, and he will be asking you about your symptoms and the unique way in which your symptoms affect you.

If you come for a chronic condition (a disease that lasts a long time) be prepared to talk about the medical history of your family and yourself in as much detail as possible. Your homeopath needs to know what illnesses you have overcome and how they have been treated, and the symptoms you are presently suffering from. He wants to get to know your personality, your temper, any changes that have occurred with the onset of your illness – be it your sleep, dreams or food cravings and aversions.

This information enables the homeopath to find the best corresponding remedy to get started. He will closely monitor the progress, and adjust the remedies according to your altering condition.

How long does it take?

Your first appointment could take a minimum of one up to two hours. Follow-up appointments typically last around 30 minutes.

Usually you will be asked to report by phone after you have taken the prescribed remedy to monitor its action.

How often do I have to come?

After your first visit, you may stay in contact with your homeopath by phone to keep him informed about any changes in your condition.

You may have to come in person for follow-up appointments as needed in one to three months intervals in chronic conditions. In acute conditions, you may see your practitioner within a few days, if phone calls are not sufficient.

Preparing for your appointment

Be sure to bring any meds you are taking, your medical records and images related to your problem. To get the most out of a consultation, it is helpful to make some notes beforehand and to think through all the issues that are affecting your health. Some homeopathic practitioners ask new patients to complete a questionnaire before their first appointment. This is a helpful way of saving time and to your advantage to do so if requested.

The Visit

First you will be asked to tell your story, and the homeopath will be listening closely to you.

Next there will be questions aiming to fully understand you as a person and how your health problem has affected you.

Your homeopath is interested in your lifestyle, eating habits and any food cravings and aversions, intolerances, temperament, personality, sleep patterns dreams, appetite, digestion, extent of sweating, location of sweat, menstrual cycle, sex, and so on and your medical history. This helps the homeopath to form a complete picture of you and how your health problem has affected you.

In addition to those more general questions, there will be quite a few detailed questions such as

- What makes a symptom better and worse? What do you have to do to make the symptom better or worse?
- At what time of the day are you better or worse? For example in the afternoon, when waking up, at midnight, and so on.
- How is the weather and the seasons affecting you?
- Are you better in a warm room or in fresh air outdoors?
- Do you need absolute rest or do you feel better when you move your body?
- Are you restless because no position feels good?
- Where does it hurt? right or left side, or ... ?
- What is the pain like? Stabbing, stitches, burning, itching etc.
- What happened just before you got ill?
- Do you prefer to be in company or are you rather by yourself?
- Do you enjoy being comforted when unwell?
- How did your mood change since getting unwell?

Detailed questions as above help to find a particular type and strength of a homeopathic remedy.

The Medicine

At the end of the consultation your homeopath will analyze your case and select a medicine for you. He may do so while you are still there, or do the analysis after you are gone. This frequently is a lengthy and complicated process.

Once the analysis is completed, he will give you a prescription and advise you how often and in what way to take the medicine.

Homeopathic medicine is usually taken in pillule form, but is also available in liquid, tablet and powder form.

Monitoring the Homeopathic Cure

You may be given a checklist to keep track of any changes in your condition while in homeopathic care.

Follow-up Visits

Follow-ups are needed to evaluate the response to the remedy administered and to adjust the therapy as needed. This is especially important in chronic conditions. A patient may feel better and decide he or she is cured, or the patient may feel worse and decide the remedy is not working. Either judgment may be completely inappropriate. An apparent improvement may not be moving in the right direction; an apparent worsening may be a therapeutic aggravation.

Chapter 10 – Homeopathic Self Care

"Be careful about reading health books. You may die of a misprint." - Mark Twain

Homeopathy is a very powerful deep-acting form of therapy. When used inappropriately, homeopathic remedies may sometimes cause problems. To use it safely, you need to learn about it as much as you can before using it on your own.

Possible problems in homeopathic self-care

- You could be producing a proving and experience the very symptoms you want to cure. This happens if a remedy is repeated too frequently and for too long.

Using Homeopathic Remedies at Home

- Learn as much as you can about classical homeopathy
- Stick to lower potencies in the beginning
- Treat only acute self-limiting conditions such as colds, and flues, and minor injuries
- Treat only generally healthy people
- Don't change remedies frequently
- Remember your limitations, and ask for proper professional help when in doubt.

With proper training, many acute conditions can be addressed with homeopathic self-care. Here is a list:

- Homeopathy can be lifesaving and minimize the effects of injuries and accidents such as sports related injuries, pain, strains, sprains, blows and concussion, dislocations, crushed fingers and toes, torn ligaments and tendons, burns, bruises, cuts and lacerations, puncture wounds, black eye.

Depending on your condition, you may need medical care which you can complement with the use of the matching homeopathic remedy.

- Acute infections such as the flu, colds, coughs, earaches, fever, sore throat
- Surgery. Promote healing and recovery and prevent the formation of scars with homeopathy
- Insect stings, animal bites and contact with poison ivy or poison oak
- Sudden problems from trauma, shock and grief
- Travel, motion and altitude sickness

Chapter 11 – Questions and Answers

"There have been two great revelations in my life: The first was bepop, the second was homeopathy." — Dizzy Gillespie

Homeopathy is a very powerful deep-acting form of therapy. When used inappropriately, homeopathic remedies may sometimes cause problems. To use it safely, you need to learn about it as much as you can before using it on your own.

What interferes with homeopathic treatment?

- Combination remedies may confuse the vital force, and while occasionally helping in the short run, they may cause serious health problems in the future. To be on the safe side, if you are considering using over the counter combination remedies, limit the use to no longer than a couple of days.

- Strong suppressive drugs like steroids and immune suppressants are No. 1 of the things that can interfere with the effectiveness of a homeopathic remedy, also birth control pills as they suppress the natural cycle. Camphor oil is known to antidote the action of the remedies. Coffee may interfere in some cases.

- A strong shock, either emotional or physical, such as being injured in a car accident or grieving the death of a close person can interfere with the effectiveness of a homeopathic medicine.

Will homeopathy work with conventional medicine?

Homeopathy can work well with conventional medicine. However, your homeopaths needs to be aware of any conventional medication you take, be it prescribed by a doctor or bought over the counter, including supplements and vitamins. There can be conflicts between the two systems of treatment, and so it is important for the homeopath to be able to identify when this is happening. No responsible homeopath will ask you to come off your conventional medication without consulting with your doctor.

In some cases, where conventional medicine is suppressing a major system of the body (such as steroids and hormone treatments) homeopathic treatment may be more difficult; remedies may have to be given more often or over a longer period of time; or sometimes homeopathy fails to work at all.

What is the best remedy for a cold, eczema, headache, flu, diarrhea, depression, etc.?

There is no such homeopathic remedy. Homeopathic medicines are not chosen on a diagnosis or label. They are chosen for a particular person with a particular condition. For any of these conditions there could be hundreds of different remedies, just like there are many different types of people with headache, eczema, hay fever, etc.

How long do I have to take a homeopathic remedy? Will I have to take it for the rest of my life?

No. It depends on your condition. In an acute condition, you will be on a homeopathic remedy until you are well.

In a chronic condition, it depends on the desired level of health.

If you take a homeopathic remedy for palliation in an incurable condition, you may have to take it as long as the condition persists.

What do all those letters mean after a homeopath's name?

Those initials after a homeopath's name are titles awarded by different homeopathic boards and schools. Homeopathic education and certification in the USA have not been standardized. There are several groups certifying their members. Any certification only testifies the particular homeopath's ability to satisfy the particular board's minimum requirements of competence. It may not reflect the practitioner's true level of mastery.

What Are the Different Kinds of Homeopathy?

In our day and age, there are two major schools of homeopathy: classical homeopathy as described in this book and pluralist homeopathy.

Classical homeopathy is also called genuine, unitarian or Hahnemannian. Its main principle is to use one remedy at a time, to address the whole person based on the principle like cures like. The pluralist approach uses several remedies simultaneously. It is prevalent in France and is used by some practitioners in North America.

Pluralist homeopathy is generally frowned upon by classical prescribers who believe that it is difficult enough to find one matching remedy and follow its effect on the patient. Giving several remedies at once makes it impossible to determine which of them is causing the change in the patient's condition.

Chapter 12 – Summary

"Homeopathy is the true and very advanced healing science much beyond the scope of current methods of chemical analysis and interpretation." - Dr. Aditya Sardana

Homeopathy is the world's fastest growing medicine. It has been proven effective for 220 years all over the world. It is a unique sophisticated system of medicine of its own, and does NOT mean home remedies or natural remedies such as herbs, vitamins, supplements or kitchen remedies.

Homeopathy is based on the universal law "like cures like", and uses a specific pharmacological method. This is called potentization. It is a special process of serial dilution and vigorous shaking of substances to a minuscule amount.

Potentized substances become curative remedies, even if they are made of toxic or inert substances.

To investigate the curative effects of a substance, healthy volunteers perform trials and carefully record the symptoms they experience. The symptoms that occur consistently are recorded and listed as a remedy picture in the homeopathic reference, the Materia Medica.

The symptoms of the sick person are essential for finding the curative remedy. They must not be suppressed.

For a remedy to be curative, the symptoms of the sick person must correspond to the symptoms the remedy is causing in a healthy person. This is called the application of the law of similar (like cures like).

When a remedy is administered to a sick person, it triggers a healing response within the individual that activates his immunity (vital force). Once the vital force reacts, healing takes place from within, directed by the vital force. We heal ourselves. This is unique to homeopathy.

Homeopathy is used in the treatment of humans, animals, and plants. It has been very effective in curing and preventing epidemics, and can be used in all stages of life for any disease condition.

The limits of homeopathy are conditions in which there is irreversible pathology.

Appendix

"Your body can heal itself. It can do so because it has a healing system. If you are in good health, you will want to know about this system, because it is what keeps you in good health and because you can enhance that condition. If you or people you love are sick, you will want to know about this system, because it is the best hope for recovery." — Andrew Well, M.D.

Links

Associations

National Center for Homeopathy has a good referral page state by state
http://www.nationalcenterforhomeopathy.org/

Minnesota Homeopathic Association keeps a list of certified homeopaths working in the state

http://minnesotahomeopathicassociation.org/

North American Society of Homeopaths (find a non-medical homeopath) http://www.homeopathy.org/

Directory of certified homeopaths
http://www.homeopathicdirectory.com

Society of Homeopaths (UK) non-medical homeopaths
www.homeopathy-soh.org

http://www.homeopathy-soh.org/research/find-out-more/

Alliance of Registered Homeopaths (UK) www.a-r-h.org/

Lots of information
http://johnbenneth.wordpress.com/author/johnbenneth/

Homeopathic medicine school / find a homeopath
http://www.homeopathycanada.com/

http://www.wholehealthnow.com/homeopathy_info/find-a-provider.html

Homeopaths without borders
www.homeopathswithoutborders-na.org

Research and Guides

Samueli Institute
https://www.samueliinstitute.org/research-areas/brain-mind-and-healing/bmh-focal-areas/nano-pharmacology

Nanoparticle study/research:
http://www.ncbi.nlm.nih.gov/pubmed/20970092

Treatment of epidemics, flu, Ebola virus
http://flusolution.net/

André Saine's answers to homeopathy critics:
http://www.homeopathy.ca/debates_2013-03-22Q1ns.shtml

Overview of "agro homeopathy"
http://www.considera.org/hrxintro.html

http://www.wholehealthnow.com/homeopathy_info/find-a-provider.html

History of homeopathy
https://www.homeopathic.com/Articles/Introduction_to_Homeopathy/A_Condensed_History_of_Homeopathy.html

Vaccines and autism

http://www.naturalnews.com/047072_MMR_vaccine_autism_government_coverup.html

Homeopathic Groups

Extraordinary Medicine www.extraordinarymedicine.org/

Homeopathy Heals www.homeopathyheals.me.uk

Homeopathy Worldwide www.homeopathyworldwide.org/

World Homeopathy Awareness Organization
www.worldhomeopathy.org/

Videos

http://tv.naturalnews.com/Browse.asp?categoryid=9

Homeopathic Pharmacies

http://ainsworths.com/

http://www.helios.co.uk/

Books

Dooley, Timothy, M.D., N.D.:
Homeopathy: Beyond Flat Earth Medicine
Timing Publishers, San Diego, CA, ISBN 1-886893-00-4

Panos, Maesimund B., M.D. and Heimlich, Jane:
Homeopathic Medicine at Home
J.P. Tarcher, Inc., Los Angeles, CA, ISBN 0-87477-195-1
Guidelines for prescribing for acute conditions, like injuries,
flus, earaches, etc.

Vithoulkas, George:
The Science of Homeopathy
Grove Press, Inc., New York, NY, ISBN 0-394-17560-3

Dana Ullman:
The Homeopathic Revolution: Why Famous People and
Cultural Heroes Choose Homeopathy

Hahnemann, Samuel:
The Organon of Medicine
J.P. Tarcher, Inc., Los Angeles, CA, ISBN 0-87477-223-0

Coulter, Harris L.:
Divided Legacy: The Conflict Between Homeopathy and the
American Medical Association
North Atlantic Books and Homeopathic Educational Services
Berkeley, CA, ISBN 0-913028-96-7

This book traces the complete history of homeopathy in the
United States: from the beginning in the mid-1800s,
through the height of popularity, and down through the
decline at the turn of the 20th century.

Christiane Maute:
Homeopathy for Plants, 2nd ed. 2014

http://www.narayana-
verlag.com/homeopathy/pdf/Homeopathy-for-Plants-
Christiane-Maute.11109_1.pdfNarayana Verlag, Kandern,
Germany, ISBN ISBN: 978-3-943309-21-8 (available on
Amazon.com)

A practical guide to the most common plant diseases, pests
and damage with information on how to treat them
homeopathical-ly. Recommended for the home gardener
and homesteader.

Publishers Notes

Disclaimer

This publication is intended to provide helpful and informative material. It is not intended to diagnose, treat, cure, or prevent any health problem or condition, nor is intended to replace the advice of a physician. No action should be taken solely on the contents of this book. Always consult your physician or qualified health-care professional on any matters regarding your health and before adopting any suggestions in this book or drawing inferences from it.

The author and publisher specifically disclaim all responsibility for any liability, loss or risk, personal or otherwise, which is incurred as a consequence, directly or indirectly, from the use or application of any contents of this book.

Dear Reader,

Thank you for reading my book. It is my wish that it was useful to you, and hopefully the book has helped you make an informed decision on applying homeopathy in your health care.

I welcome any suggestions to be considered in upcoming editions, as well as any questions you may have on homeopathy at rawfoodpublishing@gmail.com

Please leave your review on Amazon as this helps other readers to discover the book.

Thank you.

Best,

Traudl Woehlke

Books by Traudl Woehlke

Vaccine Free Healthy in a Viral Epidemic

Series Whole Health Now, Vol. 1

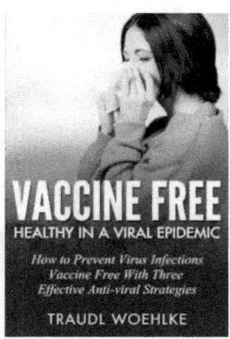

Ebooks on Amazon

Raw Food for Babies

For Happier, Healthier Infants

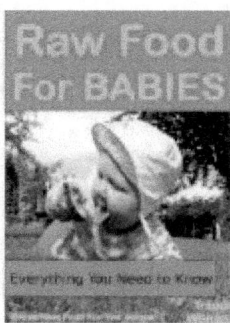

Raw Food in Pregnancy
For Easy Pregnancy, Easy Delivery, a Healthy
Baby

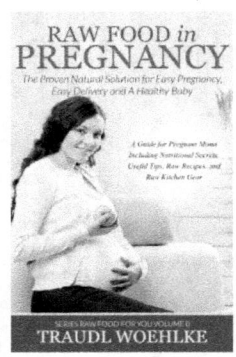

www.ingramcontent.com/pod-product-compliance
Lightning Source LLC
Chambersburg PA
CBHW071243280526
45788CB00004B/1558